To my many friends and fans…

Thank you for your love and support

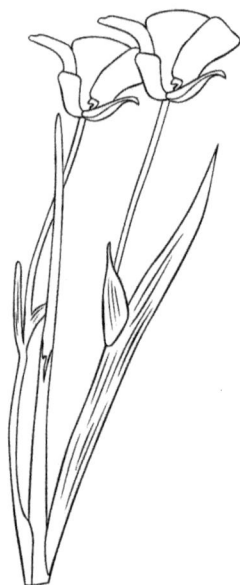

Navigating Polyamory and Monogamy

A Guide to Healthy Conscious Relationships

by
Allena Gabosch

Moons Grove Press
British Columbia, Canada

Navigating Polyamory and Monogamy:
A Guide to Healthy Conscious Relationships

Library and Archives Canada Cataloguing in Publication
Title: Navigating polyamory and monogamy : a guide to healthy conscious relationships / by Allena Gabosch.
Names: Gabosch, Allena, 1953-2020, author.
Description: First edition.
Identifiers: Canadiana (print) 20220138710 | Canadiana (ebook) 20220138788
| ISBN 9781771434621 (softcover) | ISBN 9781771434638 (PDF)
Subjects: LCSH: Non-monogamous relationships.
| LCSH: Monogamous relationships.
Classification: LCC HQ980 .G33 2022 | DDC 306.84/23—dc23

The cooperation of Stephen C. Gabosch is hereby acknowledged.

Cover artwork credit: Bloom © Pexels | Pixabay.com

Photo of Allena Gabosch by: Jim Duvall
Website: http://jimduvall.com
Facebook: https://www.facebook.com/jim.duvall.908
Twitter: https://twitter.com/JimDuvallPhoto

Extreme care has been taken by the copyright owner to ensure that all information presented in this book is accurate and up to date at the time of publishing. Neither the copyright owner nor the publisher can be held responsible for any errors or omissions. Additionally, neither is any liability assumed for damages resulting from the use of the information contained herein.

Moons Grove Press is an imprint
of CCB Publishing: www.ccbpublishing.com

Moons Grove Press
British Columbia, Canada
www.moonsgrovepress.com

Contents

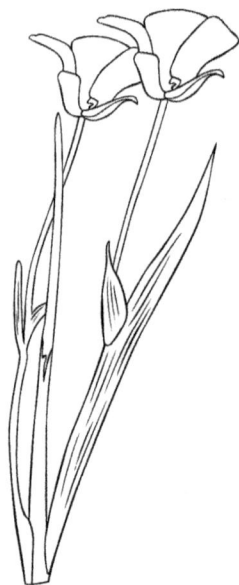

Preface

A Little Bit About Myself
and This Book

So why write another relationship book? There are already a lot of them out there (several written by friends of mine) and is another one needed? I say yes. I get requests to answer questions on Quora about relationships all the time. (**Quora** is a question-and-answer website where questions are asked, answered, edited and organized by its community of users.) I'm amazed at some of the questions. Most of the answers can be as simple as, "Ask them." This usually applies to questions like: How do I know if they like me? How can I make my partner happy? (Hint - you can't "make" anyone be or do anything. However you can talk to them about what they need to be happy in a relationship.) This shows me that there is still a lack of consciousness when it comes to creating sustainable relationships. I hope to change that with this book. I hope to bring consciousness to relationships and creating agreements that everyone can live with is a start.

An example from my own life:

My former husband Steve and I had a pretty amazing relationship. We were polyamorous from the get-go and even when we finally transformed our relationship and ended our marriage we stayed close friends. I credit that to the Principles which Steve and I created and attempted to live by throughout most of our marriage. Even at the end, we never quit using the Principles. Hopefully, you'll find all, or some, of these useful in creating a positive healthy relationship and navigating what life throws at you. I find, even years later, that I use these same Principles in my day-to-day living and relationships, even the non-romantic ones.

I am not a believer in making "rules" in my relationships; however, I'm a big believer in making agreements. What's the difference? Rules are imposed. (Parents make "rules" for their kids.) They can be punitive. They imply punishment if broken. They also can be arbitrary, one-sided and misunderstood. Conversely, agreements involve conversation and discussion and require consent. They feel like choices, not impositions. These Principles are agreements that you can create with someone (or someones), not impose upon them. The best agreements are those in which both (or all) sides feel they are being fairly treated.

Chapter 1 is about creating consciousness in your relationship. I'll explore the 10 Commandments of Poly and how to stay conscious, even when your social norm is unconscious monogamy.

In Chapters 2 to 4 I will be covering the 20 Principles to Try to Live and Relate By. The Principles were created by my former husband Steve and I to navigate our complicated poly relationship and they stayed relevant, even through our divorce. Take what works; dispose of the rest and create your own Principles to Try to Live and Relate By.

Communication is paramount in any relationship and not all conversations are easy. In Chapter 5 I will be discussing just how to have that difficult conversation: what steps to take to get ready for the conversation, the steps to conduct the conversation, and common mistakes we make when we have a difficult conversation ahead of us.

Chapter 6 is all about Happy Endings! Too often we end relationships in adversarial ways when in reality we'd love to stay friends. I'll show you how to not erase that important person in your life and how to transition from a romantic relationship into a lasting friendship.

I'll wrap things up in Chapter 7 with final tips and a few more words of wisdom. I'll talk about compersion, self-care and new relationship energy, aka NRE.

Now sit back, relax and enjoy the ride as we navigate relationships from the beginning to end.

Section 1

Introduction

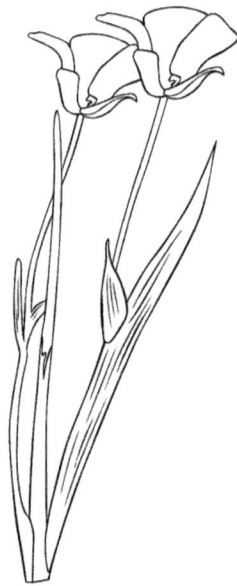

∞ Chapter 1 ∞

Conscious
Polyamory & Monogamy

Healthy relationships take consciousness. That means being aware and mindful at all times. It's important that we enter into our encounters with others as consciously as possible. That means that we suss out whether we want intimacy with someone we want sex with (sex and intimacy are very different) or do we just want a sexual encounter that fulfills our current physical needs? And if that's so, how do we make sure to communicate that to the person we are with? Being successfully polyamorous requires conscious communication, as we have a lot more to navigate than most monogamous people. That said, conscious monogamy is also very important. Monogamous folks can learn a lot from us poly people on entering into relationships consciously.

The best way to traverse the landmines in relationships, balance sex and intimacy healthfully, or just have a great fuck, is to be conscious. And in our current world, that is not usually the case. From the time we are young we just "fall" into relationships. All of a sudden we have a boyfriend or girlfriend and how in the hell did we suddenly start going steady? We add alcohol to the mix when we're teens and then we have sex with zero consciousness. And intimacy gets lost in the shuffle. And relationships suffer and never have a chance to fully form.

Conscious means having a detailed conversation about what you mean when you say, "I practice safer sex." Conscious means knowing how to differentiate between a desire for intimacy and a desire for sex. Conscious means knowing that you can have intimacy without having to use sex as the tool to get the intimacy you need. Conscious means that you can make clear your needs, wants and dreams when you are forging a new relationship. Conscious means having the difficult conversations that come up in all relationships and not avoiding them or becoming passive-aggressive. Conscious means not getting shit-faced drunk at the frat house party. Conscious means not taking advantage of the person who got shit-faced drunk at the party. Conscious means understanding what ongoing consent means. It really isn't that hard. It just means you need to be fully awake and aware and willing to communicate. That's really all it takes to be conscious.

As we delve further into our relationship it's easy to lose consciousness by becoming complacent. By forgetting to communicate and start taking each other for granted. You've been together so long you can read each other's minds (yeah right). Consciousness is important through our entire relationship.

And, if your relationship is going to transition into something new, it's even more important that we stay conscious so that it continues amicably instead of coming to a hard stop.

And as easy as it sounds, it does take work. First, poly or not, ask yourself the following questions when entering into a new relationship. For poly folks your needs, wants and dreams may be different depending on the relationship dynamic.

- What are your needs in this relationship?
- What are your desires/wants in this relationship?
- What are your dreams in this relationship?

Needs are deal breakers. They are those things that are non-negotiable. When we closely examine them, we generally discover that our needs, while essential, are few. For me, one need is to meet my other partner's primary partner. I also need integrity in my relationship. Another is safer sex.

Next, desires or wants. What is it you want in an ideal relationship? These are the things that, while negotiable, are important. For me, I want all my partners to be polyamorous. I also want my partners to not depend on me to be their sole sexual partner. This list is probably going to be fairly long and will be the basis for communicating and negotiating your relationship.

It's easy to confuse our needs and our wants. After close examination, you may find that things you think are needs are really in the wants category. Spend some time while writing these down to explain to yourself why they are needs or wants. I used to think that I needed all my partners to be poly. After some contemplation all I needed was that my partners be okay with me being poly. It was an eye opener for me.

Finally, your dreams. Those things that would make your relationship(s) ideal. My biggest dream is to live in an apartment building with all my partners, sharing a kitchen and family room and everyone having their own studio apartment. Dreams can be silly and they can also be practical. My other dream is to have all my partners get along with each other.

Think carefully about all this and realize that you are always free to change your mind and renegotiate things in the future. Relationships are not static.

If you're in a current relationship and are going through some changes, the Needs, Wants and Dreams list can be quite illuminating. Take the time, along with your partner(s) to create a list of needs, wants and dreams. I've had coaching clients who, when they shared their list with their partner, were amazed that their lists were almost identical. And that's because we generally take things for granted and usually fail to communicate clearly when we are in a relationship (especially monogamous ones). Again, traditionally monogamous relationships have traditional expectations and don't always feel the necessity to communicate their needs, wants and dreams.

Living in the Past

A while back I had a conversation with a dear friend about a mutual friend who was having a hard time moving on from her former relationship. This person had been apart from their former partner longer than they were together and yet she still clung to the past. She bemoaned that he'd moved on and had a new partner. She was not allowing herself to find successful relationships. She constantly compared everyone and everything to her former partner. It struck me that her clinging to the past gave her no room to be in the present or to plan for the future. She was stuck. And this is something that many of us do. We live in our past. We base all of our decisions on our past mistakes so as not to screw up again. We are so caught up in our need to not hurt, to not punish, to cling or to be right (or all of the above) that we just don't live.

We should not allow our past to create our present nor our future. We should not look at a potential partner and compare them to a former partner or say, "Well, they'll just cheat on me like so and so did." We should not expect them to be anything other than their authentic selves. By authentic selves, I don't mean that they can't be held accountable for their actions. Authentic self simply means what they say in life aligns with their actions, and we can't expect them to be someone they aren't. And yet we do this out of habit and unconsciously. We make up a story about what we think is so, never giving room to what's really happening. We miss out on so many opportunities because we are so stuck in our past.

That doesn't mean we can't celebrate our past successes and hopefully learn from our past mistakes. Nor does it mean that we can't fondly remember wonderful things that happened to us or miss those who are no longer with us. That is all part of being human. And that is different than allowing the past to dictate our present and future relationships.

One of the most important parts of having a conscious healthy relationship is to put the past in the past where it belongs: to realize that every new relationship is unique and different and will not be the same as the last one (or two or three) UNLESS we make it so. This means that we must enter into all relationships freshly and consciously. That we stay aware and present at all times and when we catch ourselves reverting back to our old habits of living in the past, we pinch ourselves and get back into the present. That doesn't mean we aren't affected by things that have happened in our past. It simply means that we don't allow our past to dictate our present or our future. It's easy to fall into a belief that "He did X to me so all men will do X," instead of doing the work to deal with past traumas and issues. I'm a big believer in therapy and coaching to deal with our past traumas and issues. That we stop making up stories about what we think is so and wait and see what the present gives us. It takes practice and courage, and as I said, consciousness, and it can be done. Put the past behind you and travel toward the future unburdened and ready for your next adventure.

And now for some fun. I was raised fundamentalist and the Bible was a part of my life. Here's my take on the 10 Commandments for you polyamorous and monogamous folks out there (pardon the prescriptive language, it's an homage to the original). And, I currently identify as a Reluctant Bhuddist which has a lot to do with my being focused on the present and being conscious (reluctant because I'm not great at meditation). Below is the list followed by a breakdown of what I mean:

10 Commandments of Polyamory and Monogamy

1. You shall not put anyone above yourself. No partner is better than you are.

2. You shall not create false equivalencies between partners. Everyone is in your life for their own unique reasons.

3. You shall not curse or verbally abuse a partner.

4. Keep the sanctity of all your relationships at the top of your thoughts.

5. Honor all your relationships.

6. Do not "kill off" or erase former partners. All partners were with you for a reason.

7. Do not break agreements, for that is equivalent to cheating.

8. Do not steal your partners' agency. You cannot impose your morals on them.

9. Do not lie to your partners, integrity is of utmost importance.

10. Do not covet your partner's other partners without first talking to that partner.

1. You shall not put anyone above yourself. No partner is better than you are. You are the most important person in your life.

If you are someone who is in a hierarchical poly relationship, it's easy to feel less than when you are a secondary or tertiary partner. (Those in hierarchical poly actually have a ranking system among their relationships. At the top is the person's primary partner.) Always remember that you are in their life for a reason and primary, secondary, etc. are just names not judgements.

If you are monogamous, remember that you are equal with your partner. Even if you find yourself falling into gendered roles, your "role" in the relationship is not better or lesser, it just is who you are in the relationship.

2. You shall not create false equivalencies between partners. Everyone is in your life for their own unique reasons. This is kind of a continuation of the first commandment. Even us non-hierarchical poly folk have an unconscious tendency to create a "pecking order" or rank our partners.

For those of you who are monogamous, this means that you don't compare your partner with others. Especially partners from your past. They are who they are and are with you because you both chose each other. The grass is not always greener on the other side. And it's easy to romanticize your past relationships after time has passed.

3. You shall not curse or verbally abuse a partner.

This goes without saying. I will cover behavior in other chapters. However, verbally abusing a partner is not any different than physically abusing them, in the long run. The wounds just take longer to show and sometimes longer to heal. And verbal abuse is sometimes subtle and more in the realm of passive aggressiveness than outright abuse. This can be even more damaging because it's not as apparent. That's not to say that there is anything wrong with a "potty mouth." It's cursing at someone in anger that is problematic.

4. Keep the sanctity of all your relationships at the top of your thoughts.

I use sanctity in this commandment to mean devotion. Stay devoted to your relationship(s) even when times are tough. It's easy to fall into dismissive patterns when times are tough. Devotion means love, loyalty, or enthusiasm for a person, even when the relationship is struggling. Know that the blessing of being in a relationship can be very rewarding.

5. Honor all your relationships.

This isn't just about romantic relationships, this is also about friendships and family. Be an honorable person in all relationships. This means being honest and compassionate at all times. It means not taking advantage of a person's weaknesses.

6. Do not "kill off" or erase former partners. All partners were with you for a reason.

This is hard for poly people and even harder for monogamous folks. All of our former partners gave us gifts, even the ones that ended horribly. Staying friends with former partners can be very rewarding in the long run. It takes communication and adulting (the practice of behaving in a way characteristic of a responsible adult) to avoid feeling jealous and insecure, and it can be done. And if children are involved it's even more important.

7. Do not break agreements, for that is equivalent to cheating.

Yes, poly people can cheat. Usually in the form of breaking agreements. And of course, for you monogamous people, don't cheat on your partner. It's that simple.

8. Do not steal your partners' agency. You cannot impose your morals on them.

By agency I mean that we all have the abilities to make our own choices in life. You love your partner for who they are and for who they are not. You cannot expect them to change for you. This is true whether poly or mono.

9. Do not lie to your partner(s), integrity is of utmost importance.

No explanation needed, other than "white lies" are still lies. Open communication, no matter how difficult, is the cornerstone of a good relationship (see also Chapter 5 on Difficult Conversations).

10. Do not covet your partner's other partners without first talking to that partner.

This is primarily for poly folks, and again goes back to open communication. However, even monogamous people may find themselves attracted to a close friend or someone at work. Don't hide that attraction from your partner. Have a secure enough relationship that you can talk about your attractions without your partner feeling jealous or insecure. And, if your partner tells you about their attraction to another, don't feel less than, just acknowledge that they are a human being with feelings. Of course, if your agreements are such that you don't have to tell your partner, this is not relevant. And for you solo poly folks, you still need to practice open and honest communication.

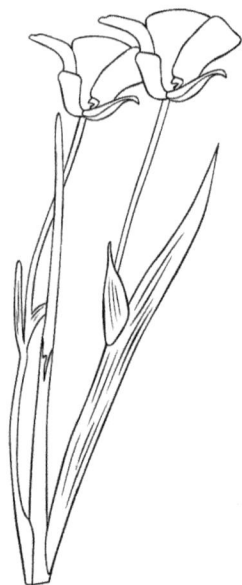

Section 2

The 20 Principles

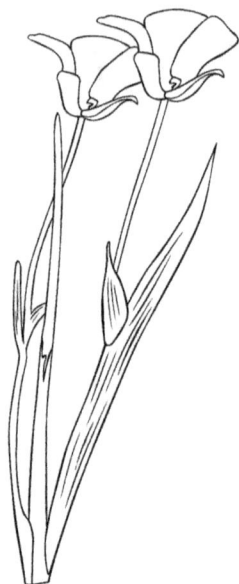

The 20 Principles

1. No surprises – (Except surprise parties and scenes and gifts and cards and that kind of fun stuff).

2. Make clear agreements on what each person is expected to do.

3. Each person should be clear about their intentions.

4. Each person should be clear about their expectations of the other.

5. No secrets or secret agendas.

6. Find ways to be genuinely supportive and uplifting toward one another, especially when times are tough.

7. Keep a sense of humor when working out differences of opinion.

8. If one loses their sense of humor, the other should be forgiving.

9. If one gets out of line, the other should be firm but forgiving, and the one out of line should acknowledge the infraction when it is pointed out.

10. Nagging is only allowed if done with humor and goodwill.

11. Never complain to a third party in place of dealing with the primary person directly.

12. When disagreeing, both sides must listen to the other intently.

13. When disagreeing, interruptions, raised voices, angry movements and demeaning language are never appropriate and must be apologized for when they are pointed out.

14. Apologies for interruptions, raised voices, angry movements and demeaning language during disagreements must be accepted.

15. When disagreeing, neither person is allowed to say, "I already told you such and such…" they have to patiently repeat themselves.

16. When disagreeing, neither person can accuse the other of starting the argument or creating the disagreement.

17. If one has bad feelings about the other during or after a disagreement they cannot blame the other for these bad feelings.

18. Past disagreements are not valid issues during a current disagreement – no "generalizing" and no "bringing up the past."

19. Short breaks from arguments are okay, however when possible, disputes should be resolved on the same day they begin.

20. If a departure is necessary during a disagreement it must be cordial and considerate.

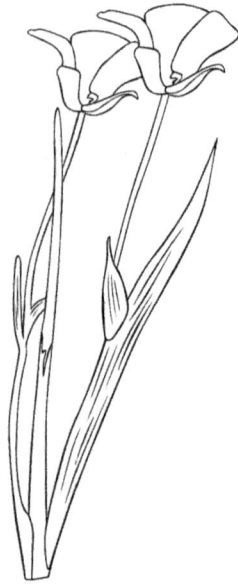

❧ Chapter 2 ☙

Agreements and Intentions
(More on Consciousness)

Now, I know that there are a lot of very conscious monogamous people as there are plenty of unconscious poly people, and from talking to my monogamous friends (yes, I have some) over the years, more often than not they still entered their relationships blindly, they forgot to create agreements and to be clear about their intentions and expectations.

In the world of unconscious relationships, many times we just "fall into" them. Remember when you were in grade school and the kid sitting next to you just announced that they were your girlfriend/boyfriend? That's kind of how it works. All of a sudden we've got a lover. All of a sudden we're engaged or married. And then there are kids. And it just keeps going. Before we know it, we realize that we never talked at all about the really important things. We're sexually incompatible. One of us is kinky. We really don't want to live in the suburbs. We didn't really want to have children.

Someone very close to me, years ago (like 40+) got married at the age of seventeen. I asked her why she rushed into this and she said, "All my friends are getting married." Then she paused, looked at me kind of funny and then said, "Oh, and I love him." That marriage lasted just long enough for her to have two wonderful children. Then they divorced and she became a struggling single mom. It was obvious that she wasn't really conscious about the whole marriage thing.

You see where I'm going with this?

Healthy Relationships Start With the First Five Principles

1) No surprises (except for gifts and cool birthday parties and other fun stuff).

This is probably the most basic of all agreements you can make in any relationship – to bring it down to one word, "communication." "No surprises" means letting your partner know before you do something that may cause them to be uncomfortable. It means we anticipate areas that may be triggers for our partners and tell them before they discover it on their own. Do you like to look at porn and your partner doesn't know? Let them know prior to them discovering it accidentally. Did a former partner start working in the cubicle next door? First thing you should do is tell your current partner about this. It's pretty simple but not always easy to do. To quote a friend, "It requires courage. It sometimes means having a conversation that your first human instinct might tell you you'd want to avoid."

It means talking – and being conscious. It means anticipating areas that may be of concern and being willing to take chances and let them know things that may be unpleasant or not optimal. I guarantee, a known potential issue is way less threatening to a relationship than an unknown imagined one. We are people who like to create stories about what we feel might be reality. These stories are seldom what is true and usually a lot scarier than reality. It's a lot harder for your partner to make up stories when you are upfront from the start; giving them the facts, even in areas that might cause distress or concern.

"No Surprises" doesn't mean that you can't keep secrets when secrets are necessary. And it doesn't mean that you can't have boundaries. "No Surprises" is not surprising somebody with an "oh shit" moment or an "aha" moment because you never told them about the fact that your mother was coming over to visit, or whatever that might be. "No Surprises" is about living within your agreements that you already have. It doesn't mean that you can't, let's say for example, be in a "don't ask, don't tell" relationship or a mono/poly relationship, as long as you're up front with your other partners about it.

Something along the line of, "My partner doesn't want to know about my other relationships. I won't be telling her about what we're doing, and she's also requested that I not tell you about our sex life, and our relationship, other than the fact that I have a happy relationship." It's okay to have those kinds of boundaries. The important things are setting those boundaries from the start and creating agreements around possible secrets and surprises up front as well.

2) Make clear agreements on what each person is expected to do.

Again, this is about communication (see a pattern?). It is the biggest hurdle we have to leap over in relationships since communicating takes consciousness and as I've already said, we have a tendency to enter into relationships (especially romantic ones) unconsciously. Communicating means being in the moment and aware, then letting your partner (or partners) know how you are, what you want and what you expect.

Take the time to talk about how the relationship is going to be constructed. Simple things like who pays for dates or who takes out the trash when you're living together should not be taken for granted. Have a conversation about this. I highly recommend that you also write it down. And, since we all know that things morph and change over time, schedule regular times to review your agreements. What seemed important early on in the relationship may not be necessary later on. See Chapter 5 on Difficult Conversations about how to be in the proper frame of mind to have this serious discussion and how to prepare for it (for example, don't have these conversations when angry or sleepy or hungry or horny).

3) Each person should be clear about their intentions.

4) Each person should be clear about their expectations of the other.

Many times, while in relationships, we expect our partners to be mind readers. "If you really loved me, you would know that I wanted to go out to dinner tonight." "How come you didn't know that I was pissed off at you for inviting your mother over last night?" Yes, it's silly and it happens all the time. Again, this is about conscious communication. Such as letting your partner know directly when you have plans or ideas that you want to carry out instead of dropping veiled hints and sideways glances and expecting them to know what you mean. And, if you want them to behave in a certain way, or do something in particular for you, then use your words and tell them what you expect. Ask, because if you don't, you don't have any right to expect an answer.

5) No secrets or secret agendas.

This kind of goes back to the "No Surprises" agreement. Don't keep secrets. Lies of omission are still lies. I'm not saying be tactless but being upfront and honest, even when it hurts, will serve you so much better in the long run. As for secret agendas – here's an example: Marrying someone who has a few habits or ways of being that you don't like with the idea that you'll find a way to secretly wear them down and change them into something more to your liking. This will backfire. If you can't have an honest conversation from the get-go then you should not be in the relationship.

There is a saying that I love. We love the person we are with for who they are AND for who they aren't. We don't try to change them into something else.

ഊ Chapter 3 ℭ

Supporting Each Other

6) Find ways to be genuinely supportive and uplifting toward one another, especially when times are tough.

While this sounds like a given, it's not as easy as you'd think. When times are tough for someone we love, they can be morose and sad and not fun to be around and it makes it difficult to be present for them when you'd really rather be out with friends at happy hour. Staying present and connected at times like this takes work.

Here are a few things that you can try to assist those you love during rough times. Listen without comment or judgement. Sometimes just being present can be enough. If appropriate, have physical contact with them. It can be very comforting to have someone just hold your hand and look at you when you're feeling overwhelmed by the world. Distract them with something fun and easy, like a trip to the zoo or dinner out: nothing that takes a lot of thought or effort, just a bit of distraction.

At the same time, be aware that you need to make your own boundaries known. It's one thing to be there for someone you love and it's another for them to walk all over you and bring you down to their level. If they are intent on staying down and want you to join them, lovingly and firmly decline. Offer to assist them in finding someone professional to talk to or to find a way to get out of whatever situation they may be in that is getting them down. We can't "fix" our loved ones; we can only assist them in finding ways to heal themselves. Be conscious that when a partner offers their support, you should be accepting of their support. Also, be aware that we may not always have the bandwidth to be there for our partner and that as long as we communicate this it's okay.

7) **Keep a sense of humor when working out differences of opinion.**

8) **If one loses their sense of humor, the other should be forgiving.**

A sense of humor will get you a long way in a relationship. It was one of the main things that kept Steve and I going when we were dealing with the end of our marriage. I truly believe that people who laugh together and those who can find the ridiculousness and silliness in most any situation will survive with flying colors. Sometimes, in the midst of a heated discussion, pointing out the irony of something said or whimsy of a particular point of view can dispel hard feelings before they become entrenched. An argument that ends in laughter is no longer an argument. It becomes something else.

Of course, there are times that no matter how silly or funny to you the situation is, your partner's sense of humor disappears. Then it's important to step back, accept that they are not going to see it your way and forgive them for being entrenched in whatever is going on. Being willing to come from a place of forgiveness during times of disagreement and loss of sense of humor can be very beneficial to the relationship.

9) **If one gets out of line, the other should be firm but forgiving, and the one out of line should acknowledge the infraction when it is pointed out.**

By out of line I mean disrespectful or inappropriate behavior. Balancing firmness with forgiveness isn't easy and it is important when dealing with issues that come up in relationships. We all get out of line at times. We forget our agreements and we treat those we love with less than loving attention. We throw tantrums. We cry. We scream. We fuck up. And a loving partner will be firm in their communication that the tantrums, crying, screaming, etc. is not appropriate nor is it furthering the relationship and conversation. And at the same time they will affirm their love for their partner and let them know that there will be no repercussions for their lapse in behavior. And when that is pointed out to them, it's their cue to step back and take a look at what it was that triggered them into throwing that tantrum. While we would like to think otherwise, we have 100% control over our behavior and no one made us throw that tantrum or scream those obscenities. Those were our choices. Letting the person we love know that we realize we were out of line and thanking them for being willing to point it out can open a whole new arena for discussion and forward movement. (If a partner is continually out of line we should examine the relationship seriously for signs of abuse.)

10) Nagging is only allowed if done with humor and goodwill.

Nagging has a bad rap. Sometimes a little nagging will get a loved one off their ass and on to bigger and better things (it was nagging that got me to finally start blogging and working on my book). However nagging with love, humor and goodwill is really just good-natured reminding. Good-natured reminding is best when it doesn't start with, "You said you would…" Finding fun and loving non-verbal ways to remind them of their agreements and the things they've forgotten works too. Little notes and even texts can be easier than face-to-face confrontations at times. This doesn't mean being passive aggressive and being unwilling to have face-to-face discussions at all. There are times when we do need to sit down and have difficult conversations with our loved ones. We'll cover that in Chapter 5.

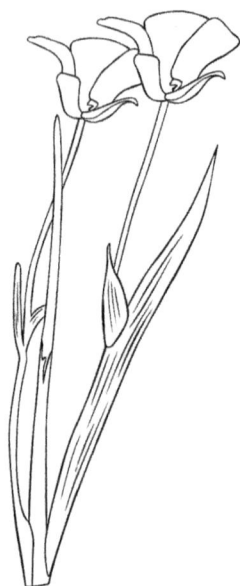

❧ Chapter 4 ☙

Dealing With
Disagreements and Issues

11) Never complain to a third party in place of dealing with the primary person directly.

No Triangulation. If you're polyamorous this is one that can be very hard to achieve. It's so easy to vent to your other partner or partners about how angry you are with a partner. This can be especially damaging when they are also partners to your partner. If you have issues take them to the person whom you have the issue with. If you're unsure what to say, then getting assistance from a disinterested third party, such as a therapist or counselor is perfectly okay. And even having one friend who you can vent with occasionally can be therapeutic. However, it will never succeed in fixing whatever problems you are dealing with.

12) When disagreeing, both sides must listen to the other intently.

This is extremely important. When we are having disagreements or arguments, it is a natural tendency to not really listen but to use their talking time to plan your next sentences. This means that no one ever really hears the other person. Active listening is very important when having difficult conversations (see Chapter 5 for more on this).

13) When disagreeing, interruptions, raised voices, angry movements and demeaning language are never appropriate and must be apologized for when they are pointed out.

14) Apologies for interruptions, raised voices, angry movements and demeaning language during disagreements must be accepted.

I acknowledge that this can be very difficult. You raise your voice, your partner raises theirs and suddenly everything has escalated into a screaming match and destruction of personal property. This is why I call this conscious conversation. We do our best to stay aware and present (more on this in Chapter 5 about Difficult Conversations).

15) When disagreeing, neither person is allowed to say, "I already told you such and such…" they have to patiently repeat themselves.

16) When disagreeing, neither person can accuse the other of starting the argument or creating the disagreement.

17) If one has bad feelings about the other during or after a disagreement they cannot blame the other for these bad feelings.

This is really about taking personal responsibility for our actions and feelings. We may not control our emotions (how they arise, when they arise), yet as I mentioned earlier, we have 100% control over our actions. No one "makes" us angry or sad or unhappy. Situations cause certain emotions to arise and as responsible adults it's up to us to deal with them as adults. That means no playing the blame game. It also means no "you made me" or "you did…" or "you…" conversations. Start conversations with "I feel" or "It occurs to me" and go from there. For example: "I feel sad that we are fighting." "It occurs to me that we can't find a solution to…"

It's not always easy. It takes practice and it takes *consciousness*. I'm going to go back to the fact that I've been talking about consciousness throughout this whole book. It takes consciousness to be able to do this and that means being self-aware. That's one of the reasons why, in the next chapter, you'll be reading about difficult conversations, which gives you a way of putting this all into a form, to make it a lot simpler and easier than just to have a disagreement or a conversation.

18) Past disagreements are not valid issues during a current disagreement – no "generalizing" and no "bringing up the past."

It is so easy to bring up the past. As I've mentioned, we live in the past so much of our time that it's often the first thing that comes up. So many times our disagreements with each other reminds us of similar issues and concerns from weeks or even years ago; especially if we haven't yet fully dealt with those issues. It's really easy to fall into the "You always do X" or "This is like when you did X" which derails the current conversation and muddies the issue. Keep the past in the past and stay present when working on issues. This doesn't mean that if there is a pattern of behavior that is damaging to the relationship that you can't bring it up (such as a partner's issues with drugs or alcohol or cheating), it just means that you need to stay in the present when discussing it. Not how it hurt you in the past or how they always do X. More like, "This pattern of behavior is currently causing me distress."

19) Short breaks from arguments are okay, however when possible, disputes should be resolved on the same day they begin.

Sometimes we need breathing room. This is pretty self-explanatory. It's kind of the old "don't go to bed angry" maxim. That said, if you need to take a break, do so. When you feel your temper getting the best of you or when you find yourself on the verge of breaking your agreements and not following the Principles, simply saying, "I need a break, please," is all that you need to do. One of my friends has a "hug break" built into their difficult conversations. At any point either of the parties can stop the conversation and ask for a hug. And, no matter how much you want to get your point across at that exact moment, if your partner asks for a break, be okay with it. Let them take a break. I guarantee the issue will still be there later and with a break from each other, solutions might arise during the time apart.

20) If a departure is necessary during a disagreement it must be cordial and considerate.

Yes, this is also important. Leaving quietly and politely is paramount. No running out of the room crying. No marching out and slamming doors. No matter how much you think it would make you feel better, it's a form of control and in some ways borderline abusive to create a scene either in a disagreement or as you are exiting. Keeping your cool is vital during disagreements.

Finally...

Here's a list of common agreements that are not included in the 20 Principles for you to consider:

If you are in a non-monogamous relationship

a) Who sleeps where – when a partner comes over does your nesting partner sleep on the couch? Is there a guestroom to use? Is a sleep-over a limit?

b) Time and resources – who pays for dinner out? How many days a week are you comfortable having your partner away?

c) Safer sex/medical issues/contraception, make no assumptions, think about what you are doing, think safety, make prior agreements with everyone. Make sure that you define what safer sex is. For one person it may mean condoms, yet for another it may also include dental dams. We never know unless we define them. Oh, on a side note about safer sex, for me, the person with the strictest safer sex agreement is the one who I follow, whether it's important to me or not.

d) Disclosure – how much information is too much, too little? What do you want to know and what would you not want to know? Some people have no interest in knowing details about their partners' other relationships or don't want their partner sharing theirs. Others, like me, want all the wonderful sexy details their partner can share.

e) Veto power – who has the right to say no to what? When I was married, Steve and I had limited veto power. It could only be used in the first 4 weeks. Our reasoning was that after four weeks, the heart could get too involved. I have no right to tell somebody to stop loving somebody. For many poly people, veto power is not on the table because it is an ultimatum, which many poly people do not resonate with. However, early on it can create a sense of security as you are learning to navigate non-monogamy. One alternative to veto power is that coming to your partner with your concerns about their new partner is an acceptable agreement.

If you are in a monogamous relationship

a) Agreements are still necessary even if you are monogamous.

b) Is flirting okay? Sometimes even monogamous people flirt, and this should be discussed early on. Make sure you define what flirting is to you.

c) Time away from each other. Everyone needs time to hang out with friends and explore things their partner may not be into. Requiring your partner to be glued to your side can be very damaging to your relationship.

Section 3

Using the Principles and Other Tips to A Healthy Relationship

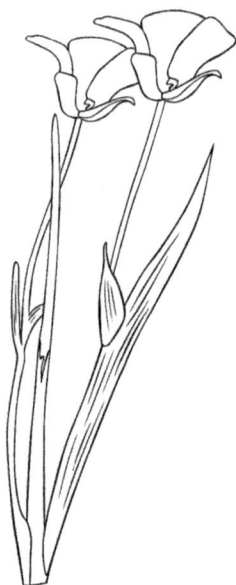

∾ Chapter 5 ∾

Difficult Conversations

Sometimes we need to have difficult conversations with those we love. If you both take the time to prepare and go into the difficult conversation consciously you'll find the solutions to whatever the problem may be will come easier than you think.

Getting Ready for the Conversation

What is the purpose of the conversation?

Why are you having this conversation? What is going on that makes this conversation especially difficult?

Be aware of any hidden agendas for the conversation. Is this about support or do you want to punish your partner for some reason? Look deeply at yourself so that you enter the conversation with good intent.

What is the issue?

Difficult conversations are usually necessary because there is an issue or problem that needs to be addressed. Make sure you are very clear on what that is and that you are not making up stories about what it may be.

What is its impact on you?

How is the issue causing you distress? How is the issue impacting you and your relationship with your partner? While you do not want to make up stories about what they may be thinking or feeling about this, consider how the issue may be impacting your partner. This will assist you in having empathy during the conversation.

What would be your IDEAL outcome?

If all things go perfectly, how would you like the conversation to end? This is a good time to begin to look at your motives for having the conversation.

What is non-negotiable?

Are there any hard limits to the outcome? Establishing what's non-negotiable up front will help steer the conversation.

What support are you committed to providing?

If this is about something that you feel your partner needs to change or do, how will you support them in their efforts?

What do both of you agree to?

What do you think you'll both agree on? Are there areas that you can come to an agreement on, especially early on in the conversation?

What assumptions are being made?

Think about any preconceived notions you may feel. You may feel intimidated, ignored, disrespected or marginalized by your partner. It's important not to assume that this is their intention. This may simply be your reaction to the difficult conversation. If you are going to make an assumption, assume that they are just as nervous and uncomfortable as you are and they also have good intentions. Remember, impact does not necessarily equal intent and, no matter the intent, actions may have negative impact.

When we're dealing with the concept that impact does not necessarily equal intent, we have to remember that both people will have their own emotional stuff that comes up. The person who feels impacted on, whether it's your intent, or not, may have some negative reactions. They may come up with, "Well, what you just said hurt me. I'm feeling very beaten down because of what you said."

So when you explain what your intent was, don't discount their feelings and the impact. Perhaps you can say something to the effect of, "I get what I said caused you pain, and because of that, I'm very sorry. My intent was never to cause you pain. My intent was to explain to you about the issue that we're dealing with." Whatever that might be. "Obviously I failed to explain myself clearly... So, let's look at another way that I can talk to you about this because I really don't want to hurt your feelings. I don't want to cause you pain." Then you work together to come up with an idea of how to deal with something that won't be quite as impactful.

Now the person may have reached that point when they say, "I don't really care! You hurt me so bad that I'm going to sit here and cry!" Then it's time to take the conversation to another level. "Maybe it's time for us to take a short pause. You need to pause. I'm going to pause. We can do it together, or we can do it separately. And let's talk when we're both feeling a little more at ease and calm."

Are buttons being pushed?

Emotions are normal and they arise sometimes without warning. While we can't control the emotions we can control our actions. Are your emotions getting the best of you? There may be a "backstory" that has nothing to do with your partner and/or the conversation you are preparing for. What personal history is being triggered? We can avoid being overly triggered by being mindful of preserving their dignity—and treating them with respect—even if we completely disagree with them.

What is your attitude toward the conversation?

If you tell yourself that it's going to be a horribly difficult conversation, it probably will be. And on the other hand, if you believe that whatever happens, that the end results will be good, then that will most likely be true.

Do they even know that there is an issue or concern?

No one likes to be blindsided by a "We need to talk" conversation. I highly advise that you share these steps with your partner so they can prepare as well. Open communication prior to the conversation is important.

If they know that there is a problem or issue, what might they be thinking about what is going on? How do you feel that they perceive the problem? Do you have an idea what solution they might suggest? Do not forget they are your partner, not your opponent.

What are your needs and fears and their needs and fears?

Think carefully about what your needs are (write them down, in fact) and what your fears are. Consider what their needs and fears may be. Remember this is not a battle or a contest with winners and losers. Look closely at any common concerns you may share.

What is your contribution to the problem?

This one is the hardest for many of us. Self-reflection. Where have we contributed to the problem? We can probably make a long list of how they contributed to the problem. That's the easy part. It's our acknowledgement of what our contributions are to the problem that is harder and very important as we prepare for the conversation.

The first steps to take

1. Choose the right place and time for the conversation

The more neutral the place the better. And while it may seem counter-intuitive, someplace that is semi-public can make the conversation work better. Maybe a coffee shop or a park will do. The library is a great place because it forces you to keep the conversation at a respectful volume. Be aware of both of your needs. Some people may need to not have constant eye contact while discussing difficult issues. So maybe a car trip or sitting side-by-side in the café or park will make it easier.

The time of day can be important, too, as well as having a full stomach. Being unrushed, well rested and fed will make a huge difference in having a successful conversation. And while it should be a given, I want to remind you, no inebriation. Alcohol and drugs have no place in difficult conversations.

2. Inquiry

Cultivate an attitude of discovery and curiosity. State the issue or concern then give them an opportunity to talk. Pretend you don't know anything (you really don't), and try to learn as much as possible about their point of view. Let them talk until they are finished. Whatever you hear, don't take it personally. It's not really about you. Try to learn as much as you can in this phase of the conversation. Be open to hear what the other person has to say before reaching closure in your mind. You'll get your turn, but don't rush things. Give them all the time they need. Listen carefully to what they are saying. Stay present and in the moment.

3. Be comfortable with silence

There will be moments in the conversation when silence occurs. Don't rush to fill it with words. Be present and conscious and listen to both the words and the silence. This is difficult, especially for us extroverts. Some people may need to even get up and move away from the conversation for a short period of time. That is an acceptable way of dealing with discomfort and a conscious way of handling emotions that may arise.

4. Acknowledgement

Acknowledgment means showing that you've heard and understood. Try to understand them so well you can make their argument for them. Then do it. Repeat back to them what you heard them say. Acknowledge whatever you can, including your own defensiveness, if it comes up.

5. Advocacy

When you sense your partner has expressed all their energy on the topic, it's your turn. What can you see from your perspective that they've missed? Help clarify your position without minimizing theirs. Be careful not to impose your ideas on them, simply state your concerns and thoughts.

6. Problem Solving

Now you're ready to begin building solutions. Brainstorming and continued inquiry are useful here. Ask them what they think might work. Whatever they say, find something you like and build on it. If the conversation becomes adversarial, go back to inquiry. Asking for your partner's point of view usually creates safety and encourages them to engage. Don't end the conversation without clear action items or a resolution.

Mistakes

It's not easy to have these conversations, no matter how much we prepare. Mistakes happen and we screw up. Being aware of possible mistakes will make them less likely.

1. Be careful not to fall into "combat mentality." This is not about winning or losing.

2. Because it's daunting to try and tackle several issues at once, we may try to roll our problems up into a less-complex Über-Problem. But the existence of such a beast is often an illusion. To avoid oversimplifying, remind yourself that if the issue was not complicated, it probably wouldn't be so hard to talk about.

3. Fear, anger, embarrassment, defensiveness – any number of unpleasant emotions can course through us during a conversation we'd rather not have. It's never our intent to be combative when having a difficult conversation, however at times our temper can get the best of us. One of the things I realized, early on, is that it can appear borderline abusive to try to control somebody by using anger, throwing a tantrum, and that kind of thing. Remember, feeling emotions is not a bad thing. Acting out on those emotions is another thing. Make a conscious choice to not act on your emotions, either by confronting our partner more aggressively or by rushing to smooth things over. Stay conscious and be calm and present. Then politely state what you really want. The tough emotions won't evaporate, but with practice, you will learn to focus on the outcome you want in spite of them.

4. Just because you're trying to move beyond the combat mentality doesn't mean your partner is. Lying, threatening, stonewalling, crying, sarcasm, shouting, silence, accusing, taking offense: tough talks can present an arsenal of thwarting ploys. You also have an array of potential responses, ranging from passive to aggressive. Again, the most effective response is to stay conscious, calm and in the moment: disarm the ploy by addressing it. For instance, if your partner has stopped responding to you, you can simply say, "I don't know how to interpret

your silence." Disarm the ploy by labeling the observed behavior.

5. We all have a weak spot, a trigger. And when someone finds it – whether inadvertently, with a stray arrow, or because they are hoping to hurt us – it becomes even harder to stay out of the combat mentality. Take the time to learn what hooks you. Just knowing where you're vulnerable will help you stay in control when someone pokes you there.

6. This is my personal downfall. If we're sure a conversation is going to be tough, it's instinctive to rehearse what we'll say. But a difficult conversation is not a performance, with an actor and an audience. Once you've started the discussion, your partner could react in any number of ways – and having a "script" in mind will hamper your ability to listen effectively and react accordingly. Go into the conversation with an open mind and be in the moment as much as possible during the conversation.

If you get stuck, a handy phrase to remember is, "I'm realizing as we talk that I don't fully understand how you see this problem." Admitting what you don't know can be a powerful way to get a conversation back on track.

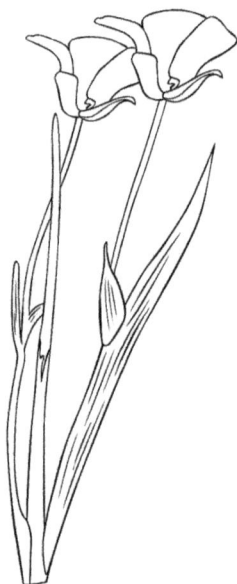

‿ Chapter 6 ‿

Happy Endings

Once Upon A Time...

There is this romantic notion that not only are relationships forever but that they happen in one fell swoop. Love at first sight. Swept off your feet. Your Prince (or Princess) has come. Etc., etc., etc. The reality is, that once the bloom wears off of the romance and the new relationship energy has waned, you can be left feeling a bit unprepared for the relationship that you just entered into. Not only have you entangled your hearts, you've most likely entangled your money, your home, your possessions and in some cases, your children. Now if the happily ever after and until death do us part portions of the fairy tale called a relationship are true for you, then the commingling of your life most likely will be painless. However, for many of us it just doesn't work out that way.

We find, after time, that our white knight is really a troll and our princess is a queen who needs to be treated like one all the time. And you never bargained for a castle in a swamp with no running water. Okay, I am being a bit facetious, yet the reality is many relationships end prematurely or at least before death. Personally, I think relationships that end when they need to end are the ones that are healthy. The length of a relationship does not determine the success of the relationship. It's holding on to a bad relationship because of some sort of misguided societal or familial pressure that creates the animosity and vitriol we see so often during breakups.

People don't know how to transition or end relationships. In our society the stereotypical divorce or breakup ends with screams and anger and vindictiveness and an attempt to take the other for whatever they can get. Seldom is there any acknowledgement of the love and time and energy that was spent in the relationship when it was going well. For some, years of happiness are immediately erased and totally forgotten.

Now I realize that there are some relationships that are toxic from the beginning or as soon as the New Relationship Energy aka NRE wears off. (See Chapter 7 for more about NRE.) I won't be addressing those relationships here. That's a whole different subject. What I will be addressing are those relationships that begin just fine. They're loving, fun, exciting and then something goes south. The relationship devolves. And by the end of it all, the fun and love has turned into anger and regret and at times a complete disallowing of the good parts of the relationship. And, since breakups don't happen in a vacuum and there is usually some sort of culpability, the anger and hurt create a breeding ground for a breakup that deteriorates into a whole undignified mess.

It doesn't have to be this way. When it comes to relationships and ending them, I've lived a blessed life.

With very few exceptions, my romantic relationships have always ended on an up note and with some I've even maintained a friendship. This doesn't happen in a vacuum. I realized after my last divorce that I must be doing something right. I've re-examined my life and while for the most part it seems to have been sheer luck and a determination on my part to not increase the pain by becoming enemies, there are also some things that I've done that created the whole possibility of staying friends and having a breakup that had some dignity to it. I also realized that I wasn't the only one out there who had continued friendships and maintained positive relationships. I've talked to a fair amount of folks who have had "Happy Endings" for a variety of reasons. Some because they have children. Others because they realize that their partner is still someone worth loving and having in their life. Others just because they couldn't dream it could be any different.

For a relationship to have a Happy Ending (or as a friend called it Happy Evolution) it has to have a great beginning and a solid foundation. I know it sounds a bit preposterous, however the better the relationship you have with a partner the odds are that your breakup (or as I like to say, relationship transition) will be equally as good.

Just how do you prepare for something that you do not want to ever happen? How do you keep it romantic and yet use common sense and create the safeguards you need to ensure happy ever after, no matter what?

First of all you set a legal groundwork that protects all parties. If you're entering a legal marriage, then research the local laws regarding property and commingling of assets. If you're not able to or don't wish to get legally married, then get advice from a good attorney on powers of attorney, common law marriages, wills, trusts, etc. Know that each state (province, country) is different and that it's important for you to do the research for your state. And I believe that for all parties involved a prenuptial (or a pre non-nuptial) agreement is very important.

Oh, I know, it's not romantic. There is this misguided notion that anyone who asks for a prenup doesn't trust or love their partner. Or that "if you loved me you wouldn't ask for such a thing." And there is the notion that prenups are for the guy (in a heterosexual relationship) and the woman always loses. That couldn't be further from the truth. A prenuptial agreement gives you both peace of mind by laying the groundwork for the future. Sure it's not romantic, it's a practical and necessary document and all marriages should have some form of prenup (it doesn't necessarily have to do with money either... it could cover other assets, children, pets, favorite toys, etc.). When ending legal marriages, our current system sets us up to be adversaries. When there is the respondent and the plaintiff, there is an antagonistic point of view. The more we can do to make the relationship ending or transition less adversarial, the better off we're going to be as humans.

As mentioned earlier, create relationship agreements between you and your partner(s). Steve and I never quit living by our Relationship Agreements, even as we were going through our divorce. They had become such a part of our life that it was totally natural for us. One day we were at a restaurant, going over financial stuff for our separation agreement (finances were the one area we had the most issues) and our conversation got heated and I stood up and stormed out of the restaurant. I got outside and realized I'd broken agreement number 20 – If a departure is necessary during a disagreement it must be cordial and considerate. I immediately turned around and went back in and apologized. Steve accepted my apology and we continued our discussion.

When we finished our separation agreement, Steve wrote a paragraph that said: *Steve and Allena agree that being together is one of the most important things in their life. And that if at all possible they will always be there for each other.* This was in our legal separation agreement and also in our divorce decree. And when needed, we've been there for each other since the divorce.

Once you've chosen to transition your relationship, how do you do it? Moving on isn't always easy.

Moving On

Letting go of the past

As mentioned earlier, humans tend to live in our past and our future and we forget that the most power and satisfaction comes from living in the present. For many people, one of the hardest things when a relationship transitions is to move on and let go of the past. How do we do that when we are in the midst of transitioning from a relationship to hopefully a friendship? It's easy to want to dwell here. Rehashing all the good or the bad. Guess what? It won't change anything. It's just going to make you miserable.

No triangulation. Triangulation is bringing others who are close to both of you into whatever disagreement you are having with the partner you are ending your relationship with (actually, triangulation, as already mentioned, is never appropriate). This means, not venting with another partner if you're poly (or a mutual friend if you're monogamous) about what an asshole your departing partner is. It means dealing with your own shit. That said, it doesn't mean you can't get comfort and love from another partner or close friend, just don't bring them into the disagreements.

One exception is to find one good friend (who is not close to your partner) who you can vent to about anything and use them as your "past regret" friend. When shit comes up, call them. And the most you can vent is for five minutes (which to your friend may feel like forever). Then stop. (I used to set a timer when I caught myself feeling sorry for myself over relationship transitions. For ten minutes I was supposed to wallow in self-pity and do nothing else. After three or four minutes, I'd start laughing.)

When you find yourself mired in the past, stop and think about all the good things in the present. No matter how crappy you feel there will be good things out there if you just look. Take the time to write them down, so you can revisit them when you're feeling stuck.

Forgiveness

Be forgiving of yourself and the other person. We all make mistakes and we all grow and move in different ways. Seldom is there truly a "bad guy" when relationships transition. Usually we grow apart or our lives take sudden twists and the relationship is no longer what it was. And sometimes that means moving on. Being able to forgive yourself for what seems to be your part in this, is the first step. Forgiving them is the next. Human beings make mistakes and you and your partner are humans. Don't make them into a supervillain or even a superhero.

Take time apart

Usually one of the people involved is hopeful that there will be some sort of reconnection and that everything will go back to normal if they just keep working on the relationship. That seldom happens. As I've said, I'm a huge advocate of staying friends if at all possible when you transition out of a relationship. The best way to do that is to take time apart. If both of you are in agreement, set a date for lunch or coffee at least two months into the future. Then meet and check-in with each other.

Of course if there are kids involved or other things that require you to interact then a different tactic will be needed. The best thing to do in these circumstances is to only have contact as necessary and to take even a few more months before that solo lunch date.

When you have children, you're going to have to see each other more often. That's just a given. So, it's a lot easier to fall into the, "Maybe we can get back together?" stage. Like I said, when there is an ending of the relationship, even if it's a mutual transition, one person usually hopes that they'll get back together. "We're going to make it better. All I have to do is x, y, z, and then they're going to love me again. And blah, blah, blah." And if you have kids, and you're constantly seeing each other, then you're going to have that narrative even more.

And then there are those who stay together because of the kids. The kids all know that you guys should really be divorced, but you stay together because of them. And again, it just keeps you in that spiral effect.

It's really important when you have children to stay friends. It's really important when you have kids that you don't blast your other partner and denigrate them, or make them less than, which people do when they are going through divorce. It's one of the reasons why I'm an advocate of happy endings.

The reason why I think that it's important to take time apart, kids or not, is that you need that space to really get that, "We're not going back. We're not going to have the relationship we had before. We're not going to be romantic again." On the slim chance that you do end up being romantic again, when enough time has passed, it becomes like a new relationship.

Nothing is forever

We get caught up sometimes in the fairy tales of relationships and when they are over, we feel like a failure because we didn't find "the one." Which means we negate all the good of the relationship and act as if we've wasted our time on the one that just "failed." You didn't fail, you lived. And living has its ups and its downs.

Nothing is forever and we need to remember that the impermanence of life is what gives us a reason to live and explore and to celebrate. Instead of looking at the future with dread, look at it as the next adventure.

Gifts

Every relationship brings you gifts. Even the worst relationships bring you gifts if you take the time to look at them. Acknowledge the gifts that you received.

Once I got to be a bridesmaid at the wedding of one of my amazing former partners. I was talking to someone about this and joked, "Always a bride never a bridesmaid," since I'd been married four times and this was the first time I was officially a bridesmaid with the dress and everything. This got us talking about my marriages. They asked if I regretted my four marriages and as someone fairly intelligent and together was I disappointed in myself for making four mistakes (I don't remember the exact wording, but this was the gist of it). My immediate response was no way did I regret any of the marriages. In fact, all four of them gave me amazing gifts.

Michael, husband number 1, was my hippy dippy guy who was responsible for many fun adventures in my life. Most importantly, I would never have ended up in Seattle if it wasn't for him.

Gary, husband number 2, was my shortest marriage (10 months). He was probably the dickiest of my husbands and yet he also gave me many gifts. The biggest gift was when we split up, he moved in with my best friend and they had an amazing daughter. (Their marriage was also short-lived. He was not a great husband, but he is an awesome father.) Their daughter Ty, my goddaughter, is one of the most capable, smart and funny women I know. She is the closest thing I'll ever have to a daughter of my own.

Fred, husband number 3, was the first person who bonked me over the head with New Relationship Energy. Never before or after have I had anyone wow me like that. And that wasn't the gift he gave me. The gift he gave me was Anthony, my stepson. I never planned on being a parent, and having him in my life changed me forever. And an added and even more wonderful gift was after being out of my life for over twenty years, Anthony came back into it bringing with him a beautiful wife, Mandy, and my incredible, delightful, intelligent, artistic, amazing (I've got hundreds of other adjectives by the way) grandchild, Jo.

And finally, Steve, husband number 4. Without him I would never have really discovered my kinky poly self. I would never have found the communities I belong to. I would never have had Beyond The Edge Café. There's a good chance that the Center for Sex Positive Culture would not have existed. The basis of this book is because of him. And I could go on and on.

People come into our lives for a reason and all of our encounters and experiences have the potential of giving us gifts. Sometimes they don't feel like gifts. I urge you to look at the people in your lives, even those who caused you pain and suffering, and see what gifts they've given you.

Celebrate you!

Celebrate your awesomeness (which is what attracted your former partner in the first place). Know that you are whole and complete just the way you are. You are worthy of love and a fulfilled life. That while you may want someone else in your life, you don't need them.

Don't rush into a new relationship

No matter how tempting, don't start a new relationship for a while. This is the time to go through the grief process and to spend time on yourself.

One of the reasons why some people rush into new relationships is that they are New Relationship Energy 'junkies.' I'm using the word 'junkie' for what it means, they are addicted to New Relationship Energy (I'll talk more about NRE in the next chapter). That's why for most of those people, those relationships don't last long. Because when the new relationship energy goes away, they're looking for that 'high' they get from that, "Oh my god!!!"

Another reason people jump into relationships too soon, is that they buy into the paradigm which says we need to be in relationships. Or we need to be completed by somebody else. One of the reasons that I highly suggest you wait a good length of time after you've ended a relationship, is so you get a chance to really understand that you are whole and complete just how you are. That you don't need someone else to complete you.

Sure, you might get lonely, and it might be kind of sad to be in the house by yourself. Yeah, you know, get a puppy! Seriously, get a puppy. Or go volunteer. Go be around people who are like you that you aren't necessarily going to fall in love with. What eventually might happen because of those types of actions is that when you are ready to start looking at a new relationship there might be people you've met that you're like, "Oh! Yeah, this is great!"

I'm not saying don't date. I'm not saying don't have sex occasionally, because we're humans and we have needs. What I am saying is be conscious enough to know that you're not going to be in a relationship with them. In other words, you're not going to move in with them. You're not going to go steady with them. If you're monogamous, you're not going to be just with them. Date a little bit.

There is nothing wrong with having a fuck buddy. There really isn't. Somebody you know you're not going to be super attached to. Or getting a sex worker, if you want to fill those needs. You can also just love you and your hitachi. Sometimes your hitachi is your best primary partner.

We don't need to have somebody stuck to our side all the time. In the long run, you may find that if you are a person who keeps falling into relationships, by taking that time, by giving yourself space, you realize that you don't need it, and that relationships are a great thing to have, but they are not a necessity. Once you get that, you become a lot more selective, and a little more conscious about those relationships you eventually enter into.

Lastly, our various communities are usually fairly small. Whether poly, kinky, gamers, sports or theater, you are both probably part of the same community.

This means that you will most likely continue to be active in your communities and that you will encounter each other from time to time. Being civil is important, being best buddies is not. You can keep your distance and still be respectful. Early on, when feelings are at their utmost, you may even want to divide up events between you to keep contact at a minimum. Finally, trashing a partner because you're angry and upset can have serious ramifications for both of you within your communities. Keep it cool.

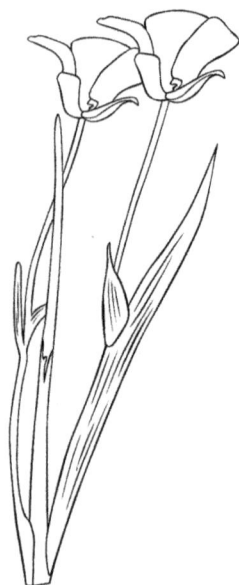

ஐ Chapter 7 ൫

Final Tips –
New Relationship Energy (NRE) &
Mature Relationship Energy (MRE),
Jealousy and Compersion,
Self-Care Is Sexy

New Relationship Energy (NRE) &
Mature Relationship Energy (MRE)

Let's talk a bit about New Relationship Energy aka NRE. NRE is that feeling you get early on in a relationship that makes you sigh when you think of your new partner. That fluttery feeling in our stomach when you know they are coming over.

According to Wikipedia, "**New relationship energy** (or NRE) refers to a state of mind experienced at the beginning of sexual and romantic relationships, typically involving heightened emotional and sexual feelings and excitement. NRE begins with the earliest attractions, may grow into full force when mutuality is established, and can fade over months or years."

I personally think it's our body's response to needing to breed and is more biological than emotional. NRE camouflages sketchy behavior and makes it hard to discern red flags early on in a relationship. We are especially vulnerable when we've recently ended a relationship, which is why I suggest waiting awhile before entering into a new relationship. Being aware of NRE makes it easier to protect ourselves from negative ramifications while enjoying the goofy feelings NRE produces. Again, it's about being conscious and aware.

In poly families it can be particularly debilitating. Our partner is acting weird and romantic, yet not with you. They can't stop talking about their new squeeze. How do we deal with it? Patience. It eventually will go away. Give them space to be goofy and in love, knowing that their NRE doesn't mean they love you less. It means that they are currently possessed by their biological urges. Eventually that will recede. I prefer what I call Mature Relationship Energy (MRE). While not as exciting as NRE, it is ultimately more satisfying.

Jealousy and Compersion

Jealousy is often conflated with envy. The two are very different: ultimately jealousy is usually a fear of losing something you feel belongs to you and envy is a desire for something someone else has.

Jealousy is a normal human emotion and it arises when it arises. Never feel bad for feeling jealous. It's not jealousy that can cause problems, it's acting out and using jealousy as a reason for bad behavior, that causes problems. You know, that "you made me jealous and that's why I spray painted your fancy sports car with FUCKER on it." (I know someone this happened to.) Actually, no one "makes" us do anything, it's all our choices.

When jealousy arises, it's time for introspection. First, figure out what has triggered the jealousy. Is it a need not getting met? Or feeling neglected? Is it the fear that someone will take someone away from you? Usually it's a mishmash of feelings and it will take a bit to unravel them. Once you do, then it's time to do something proactive.

If it's ultimately about your fear that someone will steal your partner away, remind yourself that your partner chooses you, day by day, moment by moment and that if they stop choosing you, it won't be because someone else stole them away.

If it's more about needs not getting met or feeling neglected, then talk with your partner. Be very conscious about how you frame the conversation (see Chapter 5, Difficult Conversations). Avoid statements that seem blaming and start sentences with something like, "It occurs to me that…" And, if possible, find others to get those needs met. It's not always your partner's responsibility.

The poly world has created a beautiful concept called *compersion.*

Compersion n.: the feeling of taking joy in the joy that others you love share among themselves, especially taking joy in the knowledge that your beloveds are expressing their love for one another, the term was coined by the Keristan Commune in San Francisco which practiced Polyfidelity.

I like to define it as *taking joy in the loves of your loves.* That wonderful feeling when you see your partner with someone else and it makes you feel warm and happy inside. That's compersion. Some call it the opposite of jealousy. It's also something that is not strictly about being poly. Monogamous people get jealous and feel threatened by their partner's friends or interests. Find the compersion in you. To truly take joy in what makes your partner happy is a powerful place to come from.

For some people, compersion is not easy to attain. If you look at it as "we want our partners to be the happiest they can be," it will be easier to obtain compersion. I want every partner of mine to be happy and joyful. If another person brings them joy, why would I feel that it's a negative for me? I should celebrate my partners' joys. I celebrate the fact they found someone who can go to that sport event which I have no interest in going to. Or someone who fulfills that sexual need which I have no interest in.

This also covers monogamous people. Yeah, people get jealous about certain things when they're monogamous. The reality is, "Do you really want to go to that football game? No!" You want them to find somebody else to go with. Compersion is, "Oh! I'm so glad that you are going with that person. You came home from the football game really happy." Instead of being jealous or envious and saying, "They're off with so-and-so having fun and I'm home taking care of the kids!"

I have a friend who is a young woman who is from a poly world; she was born into a poly household. She told me the first time she ever felt compersion was not about her in relationships, it was about her family. She was at a concert with her father, mother, and her father's lover. She said that she almost cried from the joy of watching her father with his arms around both women, moving to the music. That is another example of compersion.

Self-Care Is Sexy

One night I was coming home from an amazing evening with a close friend (pedicure and dinner out) and realized that I wasn't feeling that great. I wasn't sick. I couldn't quite put my finger on what was going on. And then it hit me. I was overwhelmed and overbooked. I finally figured out what it means by being out of "spoons." I was out of spoons and I had too many plans for the next day; brunch with a dear friend, Easter dinner with more dear friends and an Easter egg hunt with even more friends. I cancelled everything and decided to stay home and take care of myself. No obligations to anyone other than myself.

Sometimes we need to stop and do self-care. What is self-care? As a friend said, "Self-care is whatever makes you feel whole." For me it is a zero-obligations day (well one and that's my Joke of the Day on Facebook every morning). Self-care is finding what it is that heals you when you're overwhelmed. It can be as simple as chocolate or as complicated as sexting with someone you've never met. Self-care is when you can be selfish and do whatever it is you need to do to get back on track with your life. We all need a little self-care.

ಎ Final Thoughts ಛ

I hope that you found something of value in my little book on conscious relationships. It truly was a labor of love. I couldn't have done it without the support of some amazing friends and my Patreons. I'm not going to thank everyone personally, because I know I'll forget someone (chemo brain sucks). You know who you are. Thank you all!

www.ingramcontent.com/pod-product-compliance
Lightning Source LLC
Chambersburg PA
CBHW021347090426
42742CB00008B/766